TRUE SCARY

CRYPTID

HORROR STORIES

TABLE OF CONTENTS:

STORY 1

I can still feel the adrenaline coursing through my veins as I recount the harrowing tale of that fishing trip in the Everglades with my future father-in-law, Jim. What started as a promising day of fishing turned into an ordeal that shook me to my core.

It all began innocently enough. My fiancée and I had decided to spend a week in Florida, visiting her parents in Boca Raton. Eager to bond with Jim, who was an avid fisherman, I suggested a fishing trip to the Everglades. He loved the idea, even though he had never fished there before.

The day we set out was filled with anticipation. We towed Jim's modest 14-foot tracker boat behind us, a vessel perfectly suited for the narrow waterways of the Everglades. Unplugged from the digital world, we left our phones and GPS behind, relying solely on our wits and a sense of adventure.

The morning was glorious as we launched the boat around 9 AM. The plan was simple: fish until 2 PM, then head back home for a family dinner. Little did we know that our adventure would take an unexpected turn.

The Everglades' labyrinthine channels and canals proved more challenging than we had anticipated. Despite our best efforts to navigate, we found ourselves lost in the vast maze by early afternoon. Panic hadn't set in yet, but the sinking feeling of being disoriented lingered.

Around 1 PM, as we contemplated retracing our steps, I caught a glimpse of something peculiar along the bank. A creature, green and scaly, standing upright on two legs, plunged into the water. I dismissed it as an oddly positioned alligator, attributing the illusion to the sun's angle.

As the sun dipped lower, our predicament became more serious. Dehydrated, lost, and with the daylight waning, we faced an unsettling reality. The turning point came when I noticed something in the water behind our boat—a creature moving unnaturally fast, resembling an alligator but with an alarming agility.

Instinct kicked in. I gunned the throttle, creating a burst of speed that surprised both Jim and the creature. In the chaos that followed, Jim toppled into the water, and the creature, now standing on two legs, attacked with razor-sharp claws. A swift maneuver saved me from a potentially fatal blow.

With Jim in the water and the creature blocking our path, I made a split-second decision. I turned the boat around, accelerated, and rammed into the creature. The impact created a disturbance, and we seized the opportunity to rescue Jim.

The minutes that followed were a blur of fear and urgency. We raced through the channels, circles within circles, until we encountered a group of fellow boaters who led us back to the boat ramp. The relief of being close to safety was palpable.

Returning to Jim's home, we were met with concerned and frustrated wives who had bombarded us with missed calls. Jim, initially upset, eventually laughed off the incident, chalking it up to an overreaction on my part.

Yet, deep down, I knew it wasn't a mere overreaction. Alligators don't stand on two legs or attack with claws. What we encountered in the Everglades defied explanation—a mysterious creature that probably shouldn't exist, leaving me with lingering questions about the untamed mysteries hidden within the heart of the wild.

STORY 2

The story about the strange apelike creature that had been seen by my neighbor's friend up on Rocky Point Road had my curiosity piqued. It was a tale that seemed to defy explanation, and my neighbor's son, the messenger of this bizarre encounter, shared the details with me one evening as we chatted over the backyard fence.

According to my neighbor's son, the incident occurred early in the morning. The shaken friend had been driving down Rocky Point

Road when a creature, no more than 4 or 5 feet tall, darted across the road on two legs. What set this apart from a typical animal sighting was the creature's unexpected agility. It reportedly grabbed the top of the bank, swung its legs under its arms, and propelled itself into a swift run before disappearing into the woods.

The description was vague—4 to 5 feet tall, long arms—but it was enough to pique my interest. What fascinated me even more was the fact that others in the area had reported similar encounters. It wasn't just a one-time occurrence; there seemed to be a pattern. My neighbor's son mentioned that a few other residents along Rocky Point Road had witnessed the same or similar creatures.

As my neighbor relayed the story, he revealed that he, too, had a firsthand experience with the enigmatic being. His sighting, about 500 feet from his friend's encounter, described a creature around 4 feet tall with a face reminiscent of the extraterrestrial character from the movie E.T. Long arms, short legs, and a dark, possibly brownish, hue completed the peculiar image.

The shared experiences within the community created a palpable air of mystery, prompting me to contemplate a small investigation. Armed with a camera and accompanied by a few friends, I planned to venture up to Rocky Point Road, hoping to catch evidence of the creature or, at the very least, gain some insight into the strange occurrences.

Before embarking on this curious journey, I felt it necessary to speak directly with my neighbor and perhaps gather contact information for others who might have additional information or experiences to share. A phone call was in order—a conversation that promised to unravel more about the cryptic happenings along that secluded stretch of road.

After arranging to speak with my neighbor, I couldn't shake the feeling of anticipation mixed with trepidation. The prospect of a creature, smaller and more agile than the legendary Bigfoot, lurking in the woods of Rocky Point Road fueled my curiosity and set the stage for an investigation that held the promise of uncovering the unknown.

STORY 3

The echoes of that fateful day in the Everglades still reverberate in my mind, a tale of adventure turned nightmare that left me questioning the very fabric of reality. It all began innocently enough—a weeklong trip to Florida to visit my fiancée's parents in Boca Raton. Little did I know, this journey would lead me to the heart of a mystery that defied explanation.

The idea of a fishing trip to the Everglades had sparked excitement in both my future father-in-law, Jim, and me. Jim, retired and the proud owner of a modest 14-foot tracker boat, was a seasoned enthusiast of local lakes but had never ventured into the enigmatic waters of the Glades.

A few days into our visit, we decided to embark on our Everglades fishing expedition. The morning was crisp as we towed Jim's boat behind us, the anticipation building with each passing mile. Devoid of modern technology, our reliance on instinct and experience proved to be a double-edged sword.

Launching the boat around 9 AM, we planned to fish until 2 PM, leaving ample time to return home for a family dinner. The initial hours were filled with the thrill of the wild—encounters with alligators, successful fishing stops, and the joy of sharing these moments with Jim.

As the clock ticked past 1 PM, we made the decision to start our journey back. Little did we realize that the labyrinthine channels and canals of the Everglades would soon become a maze, ensnaring us in their bewildering complexity. Panic hadn't set in, but the realization that we were lost began to cast a shadow over our once carefree adventure.

Around the turn of another channel, my eyes caught something out of the ordinary—a figure standing along the bank, diving into the water as we approached. A green scaly complexion, standing upright on two legs—my mind raced to rationalize it as an alligator caught in an odd angle of sunlight. The sinking feeling persisted, but we had more immediate concerns.

The sun began its descent, painting the sky in hues of orange and pink. We hadn't encountered a single soul, and the absence of familiar landmarks added to our disorientation. Our supplies were dwindling, and the realization that we were deep within the Everglades with no means of navigation intensified the growing unease.

A few canals later, a sense of dread crawled up my spine. Something in the water behind the boat, moving too fast for an alligator. Panic set in as the creature sped towards me. With a surge of adrenaline, I gunned the throttle, inadvertently sending Jim tumbling into the water. Simultaneously, the creature, emerging from the depths, lashed out with razor-sharp claws.

It stood on two legs, greenish-black scales, serrated teeth, a grotesque hybrid of human and alligator. A moment of sheer terror unfolded, with the creature between me and Jim. Desperation kicked in, and I turned the boat, charging forward with all the speed it could muster.

The impact was jarring, the boat tilting dangerously, but the creature disappeared from view. I pulled Jim back on board, the chaotic wake lapping against the channel's sides. We sped away, leaving the nightmare behind, only to find ourselves going in circles for what felt like hours.

Eventually, a group of fellow boaters led us back to the boat ramp. Our phones, left behind in the truck, revealed a barrage of missed calls from worried wives. Jim, initially upset, eventually laughed it off, attributing my reaction to an overactive imagination.

Yet, deep down, I knew what I had seen was no overreaction. Alligators don't stand on two legs, and they certainly don't attack with claws. The Everglades had concealed a secret, an anomaly that defied logic and begged the question: what other mysteries lay hidden in the depths of those murky waters? Whatever that creature was, it shouldn't exist, and its existence had left an indelible mark on our once-idyllic fishing trip, turning it into an encounter with the unknown.

STORY 4

The tale of the mysterious apelike creature on Rocky Point Road had infiltrated our quiet suburban neighborhood like a chilling whisper. It was my neighbor's son who first shared the spine-tingling account, a story that unfolded like a surreal scene from a horror movie. The protagonist? My neighbor's friend, who resides far up Rocky Point Road.

The shivering witness, seeking refuge at my neighbor's house, had been driving down Rocky Point Road one morning. The exact time remained elusive, but the impression was that it unfolded in the early hours, when the world still clung to the quiet embrace of dawn. As my neighbor's son relayed the harrowing narrative, the details painted a picture that defied rational explanation.

An apelike being, mere feet in stature—four or five to be precise— had darted across the road. The creature's bipedal sprint was only the beginning of the unsettling display. With an almost supernatural agility, it gripped the top of the bank on the roadside, hauling its body up. What ensued was a grotesque contortion—swinging legs under arms, pushing into a run, and vanishing into the dense woods.

The witness, visibly shaken, provided scant details about the creature's appearance—only its diminutive stature and long arms were discernable. Yet, the terror etched across his face spoke volumes about the surreal encounter. As the story unfolded, my neighbor chimed in, recounting his own eerie brush with the enigmatic being.

It seemed my neighbor had glimpsed the creature some time ago, roughly 500 feet from the recent sighting. His description painted an equally bizarre picture—a four-foot-tall entity with an E.T.-like monkey face. Long arms hung by its sides, contrasting with its short legs. The creature, according to my neighbor, bore a coat of black or brownish fur.

Intrigued and captivated by the strange accounts, I found myself contemplating an investigation. Armed with a camera and accompanied by a friend or two, I aimed to venture up Rocky Point Road, hoping to capture evidence of this elusive entity or, at the very least, unravel the mystery that hung in the air.

The situation, though unconventional, warranted exploration. This wasn't the typical Bigfoot sighting, standing tall at 8 or 10 feet. Instead, it was a smaller, yet equally unsettling manifestation, a creature that defied the boundaries of conventional understanding.

Before embarking on this endeavor, I decided to reach out to my neighbor directly. A phone call seemed the most prudent approach, a way to gather more information and perhaps secure contact details for others who might have encountered or witnessed the apelike entity. The quest for understanding was tinged with a sense of trepidation, a journey into the unknown that promised answers but also raised questions about the inexplicable mysteries that lurked within the shadows of our seemingly ordinary neighborhood.

STORY 5

The Appalachian Mountains in eastern Kentucky held the backdrop for a chilling series of events that unfolded during the summer of 2020, shrouded in the mystery of Blaine Creek. It was in Lawrence County, along the tranquil waters and amid the beautiful mountains, that my mother's home stood as a solitary haven. No neighbors or houses marred the scenic landscape for half a mile around.

The incident occurred on a night when the air was thick with the sounds of the wilderness. My mother's old dog, a faithful companion, began behaving erratically. Barking, whimpering, and growling, he exhibited signs of distress that left my mother perplexed. No external noises reached her ears, leaving her to wonder at the cause of the dog's agitation.

After enduring the canine commotion for half an hour, my mother decided to investigate. Armed with a flashlight, she stepped into the darkness outside her home, surrounded by the looming presence of the Appalachian Mountains. A sense of unease settled over her as she scanned her yard and the adjacent creek. The usual suspects, like raccoons, seemed absent, and the night held an eerie stillness.

Turning to re-enter the house, she caught sight of it. The creature, described as an "alien apeman," stood on hind legs, a bizarre amalgamation of human and animal. Patches of long, light-colored fur adorned its muscular frame, standing at an imposing height of seven feet. Frozen in fear, my mother shone her light on the creature, and for a moment, their eyes met. Then, it began to move on all fours, disappearing into the darkness toward the mountain, occasionally casting backward glances that sent shivers down her spine.

Weeks later, a recurrence of her dog's agitation prompted another encounter. This time, my mother chose to remain indoors. Peering through her dining room window into the night, she spotted the creature again, further away and less detailed than the first sighting. Its odd combination of humanoid upper body and animalistic lower half stood out against the backdrop of the yard illuminated by a pole light.

Fearful but compelled to witness, my mother backed away momentarily, only to find the creature gone when she looked again. It was a surreal experience, etched into her memory with an indelible sense of dread.

In the aftermath of these encounters, my mother took precautionary measures. Every evening, as dusk settled over the mountains, she stepped onto the back porch, firing her shotgun into the air. It was a desperate bid to ward off the mysterious creature, an acknowledgment of the uneasy truce between the known and the unknown.

Over two years have passed since those fateful nights, and the creature has not returned. Yet, the ritual of firing the shotgun persists, a haunting echo of an encounter that lingers in the shadows of Lawrence County, a tale that speaks to the mysteries that can emerge from the heart of the Appalachian Mountains.

STORY 6

The eerie tales that emanate from the heart of the woods, the secrets whispered among the trees, had taken residence in the unsettling experiences my friend, a former forest ranger, had shared with me. Stories that defied explanation, leaving me to question the thin boundary between the known and the mysterious, between the forest and the shadows it concealed.

One story that lingered in my thoughts like an unwelcome guest was about a peculiar pit discovered in the depths of the woods. Reports had reached the ranger station of an inexplicable hole, a pit that seemed to defy explanation. Intrigued, my friend set out to investigate. The pit, about the size of a car, had an air of unnaturalness about it. However, what baffled him the most was not the pit itself but the odd contents within.

As he peered into the abyss, he discovered a vintage record player, seemingly untouched by the passage of time. Perplexed, he retrieved the relic and brought it to the ranger station. The record player, however, became the harbinger of an unsettling mystery. Despite the rangers filling the pit, it reappeared, now accompanied by a vintage cigarette case. Confused and wary, my friend repeated the process, only to find a leather-bound notebook upon the pit's return.

Intrigued by the bizarre pattern, my friend and his colleagues decided to deploy a small security camera to unravel the mystery. The gambit worked. The pit remained undisturbed, and the strange cycle seemed to be broken. However, the artifacts discovered—a vintage record player, a cigarette case, and a leather-bound notebook—were authentic and in impeccable condition. The notebook, when opened, revealed only a newspaper cutout that read, "April 17, 1972," accompanied by a single phrase: "it worked." The inexplicable nature of the pit and its contents left more questions than answers.

Another tale that sent shivers down my spine involved a mysterious child who emerged from the depths of the woods. The rangers, finding the seemingly ordinary boy playing in the forest, were met with a peculiar story. The child, wearing a simple t-shirt and jeans, spoke with a strange accent, revealing that English was not his mother tongue. When questioned about his parents, he only knew them by the names "k 98" and "d 54."

Efforts to obtain real names or any concrete information proved futile, as the child seemed oblivious to modern concepts like phones or cars. His nervousness heightened, and as the rangers pressed for details, the child abruptly declared a mistake and fled into the woods, disappearing without a trace. The ensuing search, involving search and rescue, police, and social media, yielded no results. The child, with his mysterious parents and cryptic answers, vanished into thin air.

As the search waned and the case turned cold, my friend's suspicions lingered. He believed the child wasn't merely lost but somehow placed in the woods—perhaps by extraterrestrial parents. The subsequent erasure of information from social media, redacted documents, and the taboo nature surrounding the case only fueled his conviction. The missing child became a haunting enigma, an unsettling reminder that the mysteries of the forest ran deeper than the shadows themselves.

STORY 7

Today marked an unusual journey for my mom and me. We embarked on a trip to my mom's friend's remote cottage, a place shrouded in both personal and historical mysteries. Our purpose was to bury her friend's beloved bearded dragon, a pet that had been stored in the freezer for three months. The peculiar circumstances of this burial brought us to a place where the lines between the past and present blurred, a place with an unsettling history.

The decision to bury the bearded dragon had been delayed due to her brother's involvement. He owned the property and lived in another province, and it was his duty to dig the hole. As he began the solemn task, he stumbled upon what he claimed to be the foundation of the first house in the area—a house where an entire family had perished in a devastating fire. The discovery sent shivers down our spines, invoking concerns about bad juju or lingering spirits.

This was not the first time her brother had unearthed historical artifacts in the area, including coins from the 18th century. However, his assertion of discovering children's bones was met with skepticism. The weight of the past hung heavily in the air as we faced the prospect of burying a pet in a place potentially haunted by a tragic history.

Despite the apprehension, we proceeded with the burial, honoring the memory of the bearded dragon. My skepticism regarding the unearthed bones lingered, but the ceremony continued. We read "The Rainbow Bridge," a comforting tribute to departed pets, and assured the bearded dragon that we would meet her again one day. The peaceful surroundings and the act of saying goodbye seemed to bring solace, as if the pet had found eternal rest.

To ensure a sense of spiritual cleansing, I burned sage throughout the process. The sage smoke, however, proved so intense that we had to move it to a firepit. As the smoke billowed and danced, an unexpected sighting captivated my attention—a spectral figure with a blend of a cacomistle and a lemur's face, its body reminiscent of a cat. The stripes on its form mirrored the smoky hues of the sage, creating an otherworldly apparition.

The enigmatic creature held my gaze before vanishing suddenly, leaving a sense of awe and wonder in its wake. Unlike an ominous or foreboding spirit, it radiated an aura of neutrality, prompting me to ponder its significance. Was it a messenger, a guardian, or simply a manifestation of the ethereal energies surrounding the cottage?

As we concluded the burial and left the remote area, I couldn't shake the feeling that the encounter with the spectral creature held a deeper meaning. Perhaps it was a sign that the bearded dragon had found peace and crossed into a realm where joy and contentment reigned. The mysteries of the cottage persisted, intertwining with personal farewells and the ephemeral presence of a spectral being, leaving me to contemplate the enigmatic tapestry woven in that remote and haunting place.

STORY 8

Our trip to Glasgow promised a memorable stay, and it wasn't just because of the city's rich history or the vibrant atmosphere. We had booked a room in a magnificent hotel that exuded an air of antiquity, adorned with plaques and photographs showcasing the famous personalities who had graced its halls over the years.

The first night in that historic hotel unfolded with a sense of awe and wonder. The ambiance was steeped in the echoes of the past, and it felt like we were temporary custodians of a bygone era. However, the tranquility of the night took an unexpected turn when I awoke, not startled, but with a distinct awareness of a presence in the room.

In that hushed darkness, words entered my mind—a communication that bypassed the conventional realms of sound. "I'm watching you," a statement delivered with an unsettling matter-of-factness. Surprisingly, there was no fear attached to the experience. It was as if the presence sought acknowledgment rather than evoking dread. Despite considering myself a bit of a scaredy cat, I found an inexplicable calmness that allowed me to drift back into slumber.

The following morning, I awoke feeling remarkably well-rested, and the peculiar encounter had slipped from my immediate memory. It wasn't until my mom, my room companion, shared her own experience at breakfast that the events of the night before resurfaced.

With a mix of incredulity and sincerity, she recounted, "You all aren't going to believe me, but I swear someone was in our room last night. I remember thinking, 'Just be still and let them finish whatever they're doing.'" Her words triggered a vivid recollection of my own nocturnal encounter, and the realization hit that something otherworldly had unfolded in our room.

The fact that both my mom and I had distinct, independent experiences within the same room added a layer of confirmation to the unearthly events. It wasn't just a figment of imagination or a shared illusion; there was an undeniable presence in that historic hotel.

Curiosity and a sense of wonder overcame me, and before we checked out, I approached the hotel staff. With a knowing smile, they acknowledged our inquiry, "Not sure, but you're not the first to mention this." The nonchalant response hinted at a well-kept secret, a shared understanding among the staff that the hotel held more than just the echoes of its illustrious past.

As we bid farewell to Glasgow and the enigmatic hotel, I couldn't help but ponder the mysteries that lingered within its walls. It was a place where the boundaries between the living and the spectral seemed to blur, leaving us with an indelible imprint of an encounter that defied explanation. The historic hotel had become more than just a temporary residence; it was a chapter in our lives woven with the threads of the inexplicable.

STORY 9

The remote Pacific island hung in the middle of the ocean like a forgotten secret, shrouded in thick jungle and ominous mystery. My team, a group of elite Navy SEALs, had been dispatched to investigate a series of perplexing disappearances that had turned the idyllic paradise into a nightmare.

As we delved deeper into the dense foliage, our mission took an unexpected turn. The abandoned military installation we discovered hinted at a sinister truth – genetic manipulation experiments aimed at creating superhuman soldiers. The island had become a breeding ground for cryptids, nightmarish human-animal hybrids with deadly skills and heightened instincts.

The oppressive air and scorching sun had already taken a toll on our squad, but we pressed on, determined to unravel the horrors that lurked within the jungle. The evidence within the dilapidated facility painted a gruesome picture, revealing the consequences of unethical experimentation gone awry.

The cryptids were relentless, stealthy predators picking off my comrades one by one. Their screams echoed through the trees, fueling my determination to survive and expose the truth behind this nightmarish experiment. Adaptation became our only option, and we fought back with the skills that had earned us the title of the best of the best.

As my squad dwindled, I found myself alone, forced to hide and wait for the backup we had desperately called for. Days turned into weeks, and my surroundings became both ally and enemy. I scavenged for survival essentials, closely observing the cryptids, hoping to identify weaknesses that could tip the scales in my favor.

In a stroke of fortune, or perhaps fate, I stumbled upon a hidden room within the remnants of the facility. Inside, a journal belonging to the lead scientist revealed the horrifying truth about the cryptids. They were once human, transformed into monsters by the very experiments we sought to expose. The island was their testing ground turned prison, and the last entry in the journal shattered my hopes – the project had been abandoned, and no rescue was imminent.

Alone and surrounded by death, I refused to succumb to despair. Armed with newfound knowledge, I continued my solitary fight against the cryptids, seeking a way to end the nightmare that had claimed my brothers in arms. The jungle became my ally as I navigated its dangers, my determination unbroken despite the overwhelming odds.

As the sole survivor of a mission gone horribly wrong, I knew backup would never come. Still, I clung to the hope that justice could be served. The cryptids had taken my comrades, but they wouldn't take me without a fight. I bided my time in the shadows, preparing for the day when I could expose the truth to the world and bring an end to the twisted experiments that had ravaged the island.

STORY 10

Working as a park ranger in the remote wilderness was a dream job, surrounded by the breathtaking beauty of nature. However, the tranquility of the wild began to unravel, replaced by an unsettling feeling that I was not alone. Strange occurrences cast a shadow over the picturesque landscapes, making me question the safety of the solitude.

On the third day, an eerie incident marked the beginning of my unease. Footsteps echoed behind me as I walked along the trail. I turned, expecting to see a fellow ranger, but the forest stood silent. I shrugged off the unease, attributing it to an overactive imagination. However, the next disturbance hit closer to home. Returning to my cabin, I discovered my supplies had been tampered with, stirring a sense of vulnerability.

As the days passed, the atmosphere in the wilderness grew more ominous. A dark figure lurked in the shadows, elusive and enigmatic. Its presence was felt rather than seen, an unsettling awareness that I was being watched. My instincts screamed at me to run, yet I forced composure upon myself, determined to unravel the mystery.

With each passing day, the feeling of being stalked intensified. Vigilance became my constant companion, overshadowing the natural beauty around me. The nights amplified the paranoia – every rustle of leaves became a potential threat. On the seventh day, the forest revealed its true nature.

While patrolling the campground, an unearthly growl shattered the silence. I strained to locate the source, only to feel an unseen presence brushing past me. Panic set in as the predator closed in, its growl echoing closer with every passing moment. Turning around, I came face to face with a massive creature, its eyes glowing malevolently in the darkness.

A creature beyond explanation pinned me to the ground with incredible strength. Its features were a blur – a thick, muscular body, razor-sharp claws, and a menacing presence. Fueled by adrenaline, I fought against the unseen assailant. Abruptly, it vanished, leaving me bruised and bewildered.

Dragging myself back to the cabin, I summoned help, recounting a tale that baffled the rescue team. They struggled to comprehend my experience, but I knew what I had encountered. An unknown predator, stalking me with an intelligence and malevolence beyond comprehension. Even now, as the years pass, the memory of that night haunts me. The wilderness, once a sanctuary, now holds a dark secret – a predator that shouldn't exist, an elusive entity that turned the beauty of nature into a nightmarish hunt.

STORY 11

It was a chilly October night in 2003, and I was driving home with my younger brother and a friend. My brother was sound asleep in the back seat, and my friend occupied the passenger seat next to me. The road stretched ahead, surrounded by the darkness of the night.

As we cruised along, our eyes were fixed on the road, alert for any signs of wildlife. Suddenly, my friend gasped, "Deer!" Her voice carried a hint of urgency, and I instinctively slowed down. We all knew the potential danger of deer darting across the road, and caution became our priority.

However, this encounter was far from ordinary. The creature we encountered was unlike any deer. It moved with an unnatural speed, almost matching the pace of our car traveling at 5 to 10 miles per hour. Perplexed, we observed its movements, expecting the typical up-and-down motion of a galloping deer. Yet, this mysterious being maintained a steady, horizontal trajectory.

As we continued to watch, a peculiar smell permeated the air. It was a bizarre amalgamation of decaying timber and the stench of a deceased animal. The scent added an eerie layer to the already strange encounter, heightening our senses.

The night offered some illumination through the moonlight, and I had my bright headlights on. If it were a deer or an elk, their light brown fur or antlers would have been visible. But all we could discern was a dark figure with a set of eyes, glowing in the headlights.

The encounter left us unnerved and puzzled. The creature's movements defied the logic of known wildlife, and its features remained shrouded in darkness. As we drove away, the mysterious encounter lingered in our minds, an unexplained enigma that defied the rational explanations we sought. We shared a collective sense of awe and uncertainty, knowing that the night had revealed something beyond the ordinary, something that defied the natural order of the world.